Too Cute To Poop

A Parent's Guide to Relieving Constipation in Babies

By Angela Knight

I0435567

Legal Disclaimer

The recommendations within this book are not medical guidelines but are for educational purposes only. You must not rely on the information in this book as an alternative to medical advice from your doctor or other professional healthcare provider.

If you have any specific questions about any medical matter, you should consult your doctor or other professional healthcare provider. If you think your child may be suffering from any medical condition, you should seek immediate medical attention.

You should never delay seeking medical advice, disregard medical advice or discontinue medical treatment because of information in this book.

Table of Contents

Introduction

The Ins and Outs of Poop

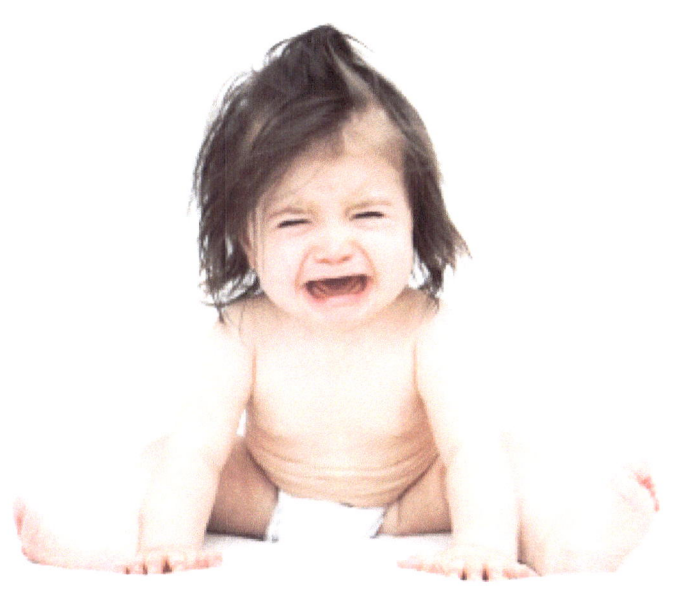

It's amazing how much time parents spend discussing the contents of their baby's nappy. Is she pooping enough? Too much? Is it the right kind, colour, texture? Doctors probably get asked more questions about baby bowel movements than almost any other baby subject! As a mother, I have dealt with constipation in babies many times and have treated it at home quite successfully. During the process of treating my son's constipation, I learnt a lot about its causes and treatments through reading, online research and talking to doctors.

When we (as adults) think of constipation, we think of not being able to go to the bathroom. With baby constipation, we are really talking about the consistency of the stool rather than how frequently they go. How do you know if they are constipated? The stool will be painful and hard to pass. Let's face it; we all know when our babies are trying to go! We also know when they are in pain from trying.

Constipation is a common concern for many parents. The frequency of bowel movements in infants varies greatly. Some infants will go after every feeding, others every four days. Both situations are normal. In general, most breastfed infants will move their bowels more often than formula-fed babies. However, if an infant has not had a bowel movement in more than four days, it is a good idea to let your doctor know, even though this can still be normal.

Because there is so much variation in how frequently an infant has a bowel movement, it is often more helpful to diagnose constipation based on other findings. For example, an infant's stool should be soft. Sometimes a hard stool may be painful for infants, and parents will report that their child is in discomfort when having a bowel movement. This is different than "straining," which is actually very common in infants. If your child seems to be straining to have a bowel movement, but the stool is soft, it is unlikely that he / she is constipated.

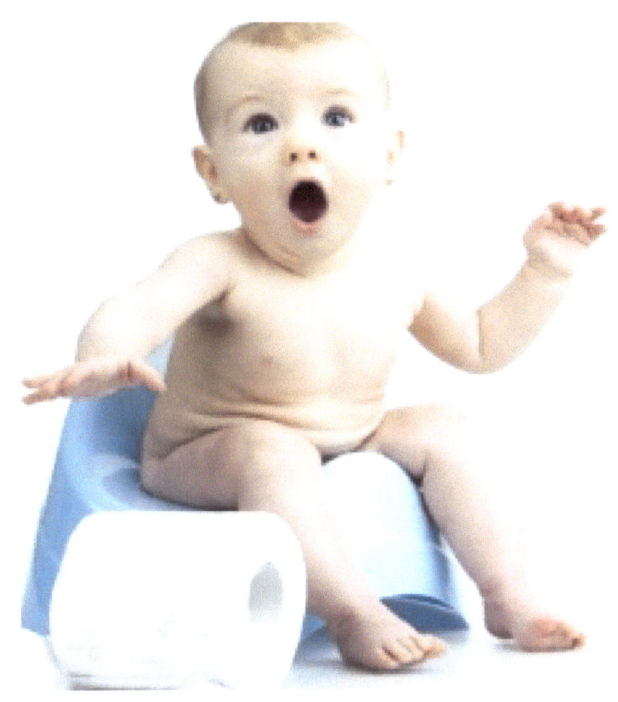

There is no medical harm if stool stays in the body for a long time, and how often your baby has bowel movements does not really define true constipation. If your baby has soft, easy-to-pass stools every 4-5 days, he / she is probably OK. On the other hand, if he / she has a hard time making bowel movements, has hard stools, has bloody or black stools, seems uncomfortable, or doesn't have a bowel movement at least once every 5 days, you should talk to your doctor.

9 Ways to Tell If Your Baby Is Constipated

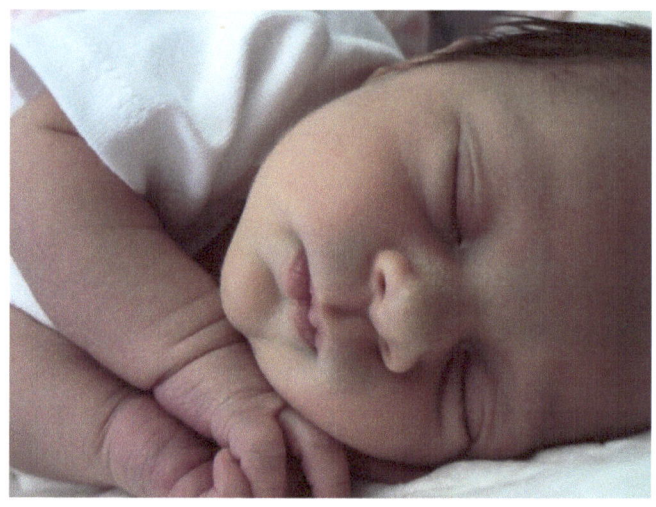

When it comes to a baby's bowel movements, there's no "normal" number or schedule — only what's normal for your baby. Your baby may pass a stool after every feeding, or wait a day or more between bowel movements. The pattern depends on what he / she eats and drinks, how active he / she is, and how quickly he / she digests food and then gets rid of waste. With practice, you'll be able to tune in to your baby's unique habits. Once you get used to the regularity of your baby's bowel movements, you will usually notice if the pattern changes.

You may notice your baby "straining" when having a bowel movement or passing gas. Parents also associate this with constipation, but that is not always the case. Straining, grunting and groaning are common, especially around 4-6 weeks of age. Your baby is becoming aware of his / her body sensations.

As your baby strains, he / she is learning which muscles do what and how to poop. The straining will decrease once he / she becomes a pooping expert. However, if your baby cries while straining, there is a problem.

The 3 Core Symptoms

Babies are usually NOT constipated unless they experience all of the following 3 signs...

1. No bowel movement in three days (for bottle-fed babies) or one week (for breastfed babies)

2. Firm, dry, pebbly stools.

3. Crying while having a bowel movement.

Other Tell-tale Signs

It's best to familiarize yourself with the full spectrum of symptoms. Any quick drawing-up of the legs, accompanied by a red faced grunting as baby attempts to have a bowel movement is a sure sign that he / she may be constipated. But constipation may also be a result or cause of other conditions so always look out for other signs that all is not well:

1. Loss of appetite

2. Apparent cramping

3. Abdominal pain

4. Evidence of dehydration, e.g. infrequent urination, sunken eyes or doughy skin.

5. Watch for any signs of blood in the stool or on the diaper. A small tear in the sensitive rectal wall may have occurred from baby forcing the passage of hard stool.

6. Strangely a very liquid poo can be also be a sign of constipation. Liquid poo can slip past the blockage of hard poo in the lower intestine. If you see this, don't assume it's diarrhoea – it may be evidence of constipation.

Breastfed vs. Bottle-fed Babies

Breastfed babies have several helpful types of bacteria in their large intestine that are capable of breaking down some of the otherwise indigestible carbohydrates, proteins and fats in milk. As a result, their stools are softer, making bowel movements easier. Breast milk also contains a hormone called motilin that increases the movement of the baby's bowels, helping them to empty. Further protection against constipation comes from the fact that a breastfed baby can draw as much milk as they need from the breasts.

For breastfed babies, normal infant stool is soft or runny. It is yellow or mustard to orange with little white flecks that look like seeds. The frequency can vary from every feed to once or twice a week. Breastfed babies are rarely constipated because breast milk is almost 100% completely digested. Many breastfed babies do have infrequent bowel movements; however this does not mean that they are constipated.

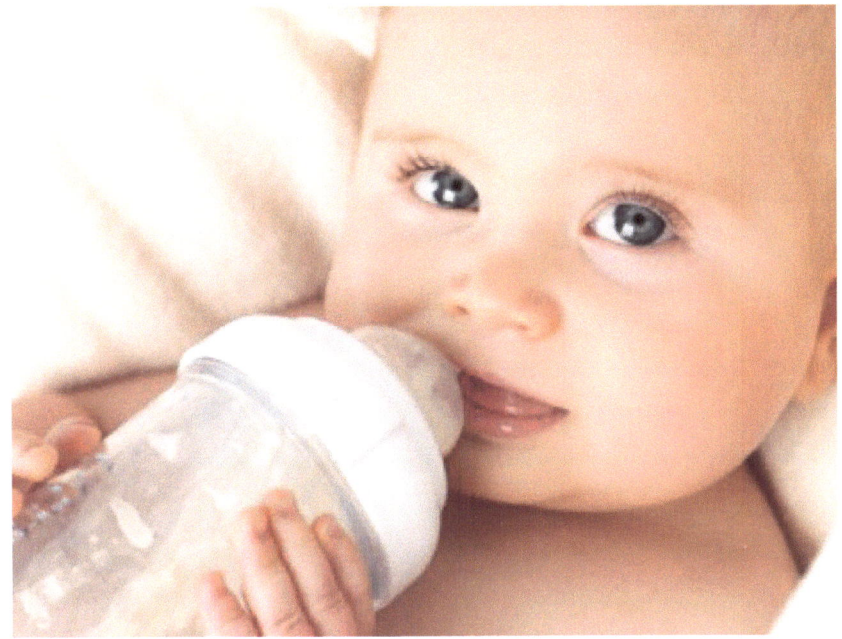

For bottle-fed babies, normal infant stool is soft paste. The colour is greyish green, yellow, tan or brown depending on the type of formula. The frequency is once or twice every 1-2 days. Formula fed babies usually battle constipation more often. This is because formula is not as easily digested and used by a baby's body.

Bowel Movements in Older Babies (from four months old)

Once a baby starts on transition foods or solids (i.e. weaning), the frequency of bowel movements and the consistency and appearance of their stools will depend on the food they eat. Your baby's stools will begin to look a bit more like ordinary stools in consistency and smell. Once your baby starts eating solid food, the pattern in bowel movements will change. Your infant will have movements several times a day or as infrequently as once every two to three days.

At this point, some babies may get slightly constipated. This is because the intestines have to get used to the new composition of the nutrients and may need a higher fluid intake to deal with some foods, such as fibrous root vegetables like carrots.

The Top 5 Causes of Infant Constipation

1. Dehydration

Your baby may be refusing milk because he / she is teething, has thrush, a throat infection, a cold, or an ear infection. Or your baby may not be drinking enough milk or water with solid foods. Whatever the reason, if your baby isn't getting enough fluids, he / she may become dehydrated and this can lead to constipation.

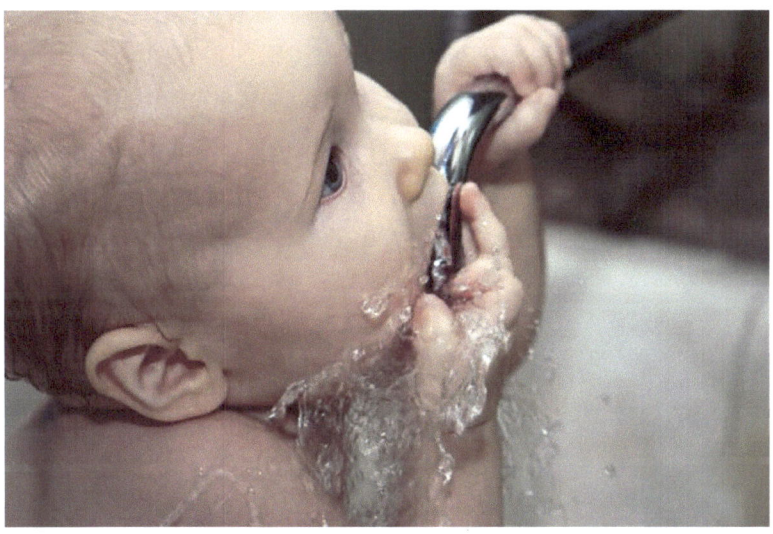

The colon will steal water from the waste material and give it to the body, causing the stools to be water deprived and hard. If a breastfed baby is a little dehydrated or dry, he or she can usually simply take more milk; unlike a bottle-fed baby who can drink no more than what is in the bottle. Once a baby's food consists of more solid food, constipation can typically be caused by dehydration.

2. Formula

Formula fed babies are more at risk of becoming constipated than breastfed babies. Certain formulas such as lactose-free or thickened formulas can be more constipating for some babies. Switching formula can also lead to constipation. If the new-born is being fed an iron-fortified formula, the temptation is to change to a formula without iron, but recent studies have shown that babies on formula without iron get constipated just as often as babies on iron-fortified formulas. So, do not discontinue the iron-fortified formula.

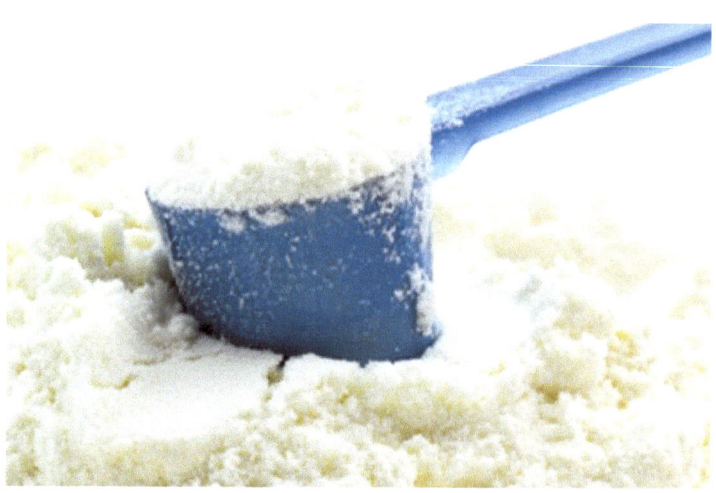

Consider the formula being offered to your baby. Some formulas are easier to digest than others. Try offering a different formula if your baby appears to be having problems digesting his / her current formula. Discuss the possibility of switching formula with your health care provider prior to doing so to be certain that you are picking the correct formula for your baby.

Keep an eye on your baby's bowel movements for several days after birth. Baby's bowel movements should pass from meconium to stool after the 3rd day of birth. If your baby continues to pass meconium or if her bowel movements remain irregular, your baby may not be getting a sufficient amount of nutrition.

3. New Foods

Don't be surprised if your baby becomes mildly constipated as he / she steps up to solid food. That's often because rice cereal, usually the first food given during this transition period, is low in fibre.

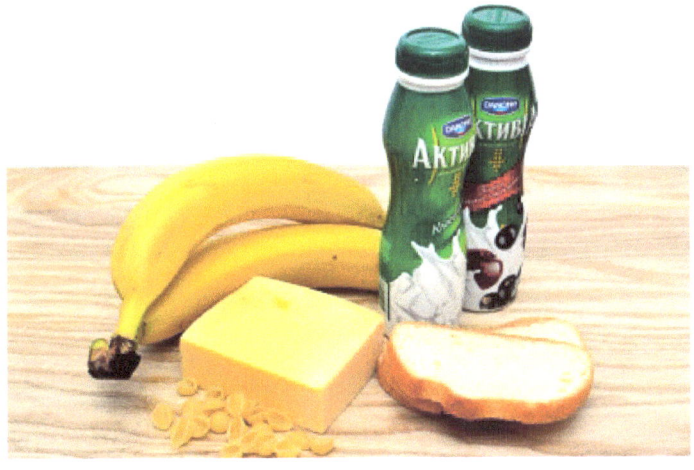

For breastfed babies, it is common to experience constipation when solid foods are first introduced into the diet or if he / she is switched from breast milk to infant formula. This is because his / her body is not used to digesting anything other than breast milk. Make sure you introduce new foods slowly to allow time for him / her to adjust. Some foods such as cheese, ice-cream, yogurt, white bread, spaghetti, bananas, corn and potatoes are known to cause constipation. Small amounts of these foods are usually not a problem.

4. Medical Condition or Illness

Occasionally, constipation can be a symptom of a food allergy, food poisoning (such as botulism), or a problem with the way the body absorbs food, known as a metabolic disorder. Very rarely, constipation in babies can be caused by congenital conditions. These can include a disease where the large intestine doesn't function properly (Hirschsprung's disease), a condition where the anus and rectum have not formed properly (anorectal malformation), spina bifida and cystic fibrosis.

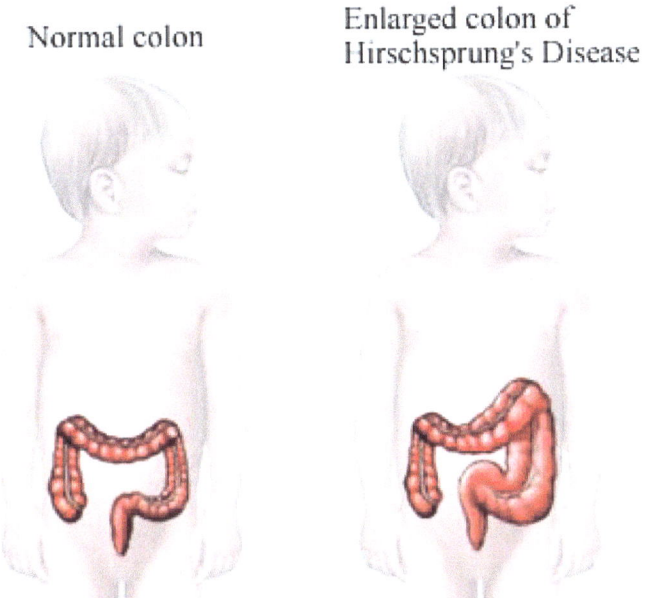

Normal colon

Enlarged colon of Hirschsprung's Disease

Normally, as digested food travels down the intestines, water and nutrients are absorbed and the waste material becomes stools. For a soft stool to form, enough water must remain in the waste material, and the lower intestinal and rectal muscles must contract and relax to move the stool along and out. A malfunction of either of these mechanisms, or poor muscle movement, can cause constipation.

The first poops that come out of a new-born are the thick, sticky, tarry meconium stools. The new-born infant should have his or her first stool within 24 hours after birth. Failure to pass stool by 48 hours of life may signify a more serious condition. Further evaluation of the infant is needed if no bowel movement has occurred within the first 48 hours.

5. Self-Perpetuating Circumstances

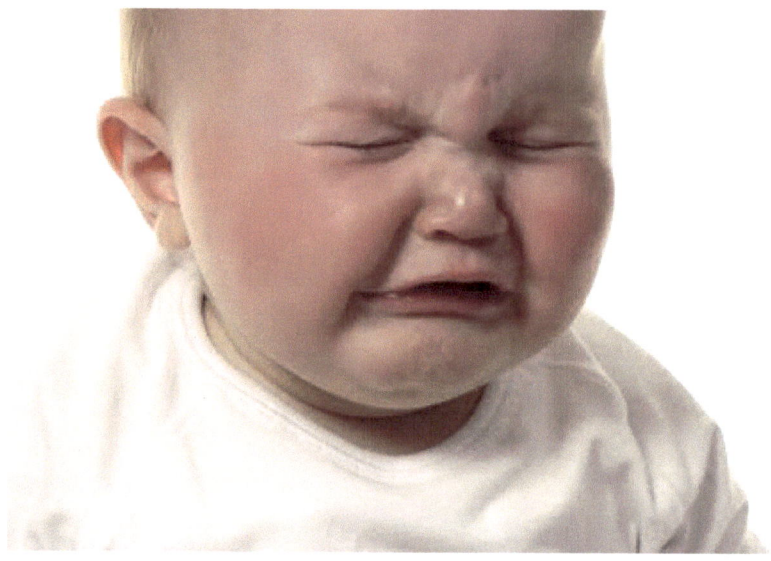

Hard stools cause pain on passage; consequently, the child holds on. The longer the stool remains, the harder it becomes – which makes it even more painful to pass. And the longer the large stool stretches the intestines, the weaker their muscle tone becomes. To complicate matters, passage of a hard stool through a narrow rectum often tears the rectal wall (called a rectal fissure), accounting for the streaks of blood. This painful tear prompts baby even more not to want to have a bowel movement.

If your baby is passing such hard, dry stools that he / she tears the delicate skin near the opening of her anus, you can apply some aloe vera lotion to the area to help it heal. Be sure to mention the tears to your baby's doctor.

The 10 Best Ways to Relieve Infant Constipation

Try not to worry too much if your baby becomes constipated. It's likely to happen now and then. One important thing to remember is to keep the baby active. Low activity levels can lead to constipation. Offer toys that roll or move. These can help encourage the baby to roll over or crawl more frequently, increasing the baby's activity level. Get down at the baby's level and play to encourage movement.

1. Baby Massage

This is a fulfilling way to nurture your child. It aids digestion, relieves colic, eases tension, regulates breathing, and spurs growth. To help your baby's bowels move, try the "I love you" technique.

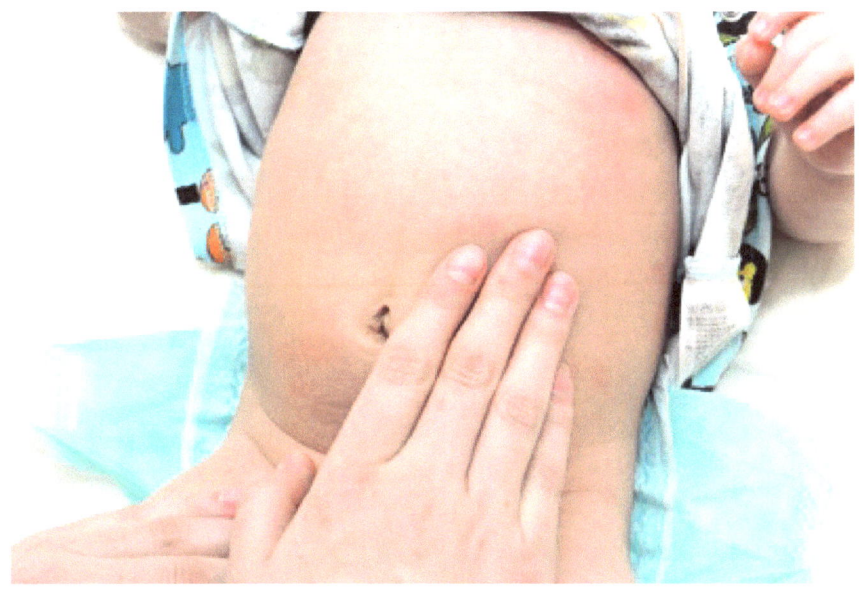

With I L U in mind, start at bottom right of baby's abdomen and using small, gentle circular movements, gently rub toward top right, forming the letter I. Stop when you feel the rib cage. Repeat this action but then move across abdomen immediately above belly button toward left side, forming the letter L. Repeat this action and then go down toward bottom left to form the letter U. Repeat 5-10 times entire I love you massage. Only continue if your baby enjoys the massage and is comfortable and relaxed.

2. Bicycle Exercise

Cycle" baby's legs which causes the stomach muscles to move and puts gentle pressure on the intestines.

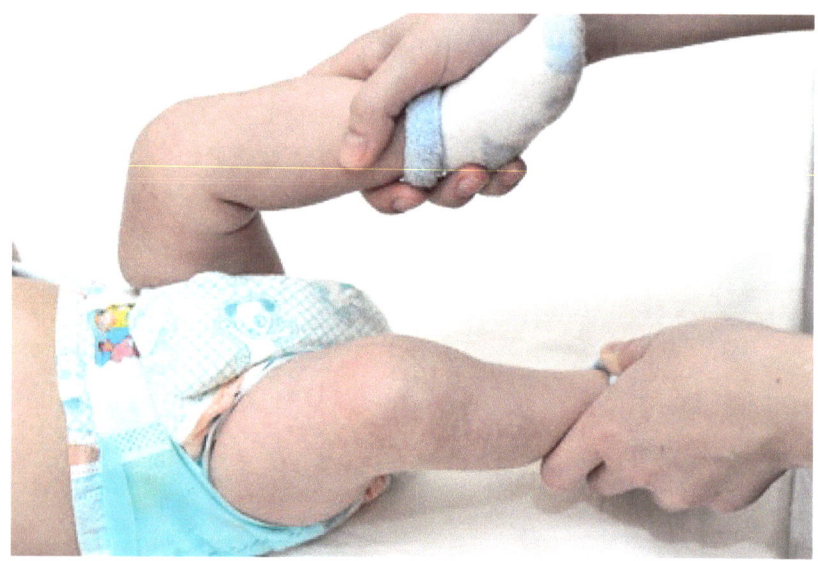

To cycle baby's legs:

1. Lay him on his back
2. Grasp his feet

3. Turn his legs in a quick but gentle cycling motion.

Do listen to your baby and stop doing this if they object or become upset by it – getting upset will aggravate the constipation. If you want to do something when babies grunt, push, or strain, try picking them up to get gravity to help them in their efforts, or try holding the knees against the chest to help them "squat" — the natural poop position.

3. Warm Bath

A warm bath can help to relax babies and make it easier for them to go. If a baby has already had a difficult movement they can become anxious about going again which can drag out the problem. Getting them to relax can really help. If you have time, energy and a spare pair of hands (to help you get baby safely in and out), get into the bath with your baby – it is a combination they love and it will help them feel very warm and comforted. When your baby is relaxed in the bath, massage baby's abdomen and get ready for the mudslide!

4. Water

Dehydration can cause or exacerbate constipation. Offer a bottle or the breast frequently to keep up the baby's fluid intake, especially during warm weather. For infants older than 2 months, give them 2 to 4 ounces of water twice a day in addition to their usual fluid intake. Keep the baby at a comfortable temperature to reduce fluid loss through perspiration. Don't overdress the baby or allow the baby to sleep and play in a hot room.

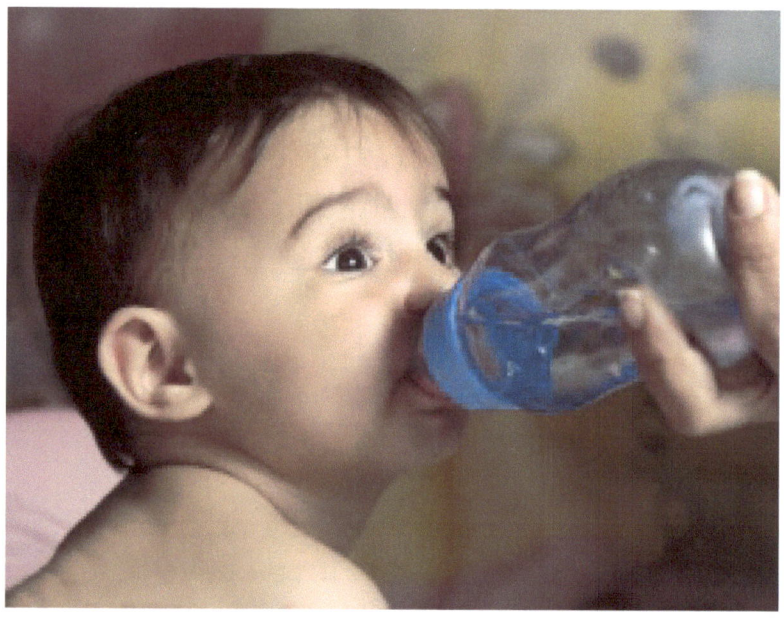

Many parents find their babies develop constipation on sun holidays – even when they are kept in the shade. Try giving them a small amount of cooled, boiled water once or twice a day – not more than 1-2oz (30-60mls) a day for babies under six months. If you give more water than this, babies will not be thirsty enough to take the right amount of feed. You may need to give more fluid than this if you are in a hot country. Once your infant gets some water it should make going to the bathroom much easier.

5. Breast Feeding

As little as ten to fifteen years ago, it was almost unheard of for a breastfed baby to be constipated. In fact, the baby books at that time almost universally stated that breastfed babies don't get constipated. Nowadays, however, this situation is becoming more commonplace and the continuing decline in the quality of the diet of nursing mothers is a likely reason.

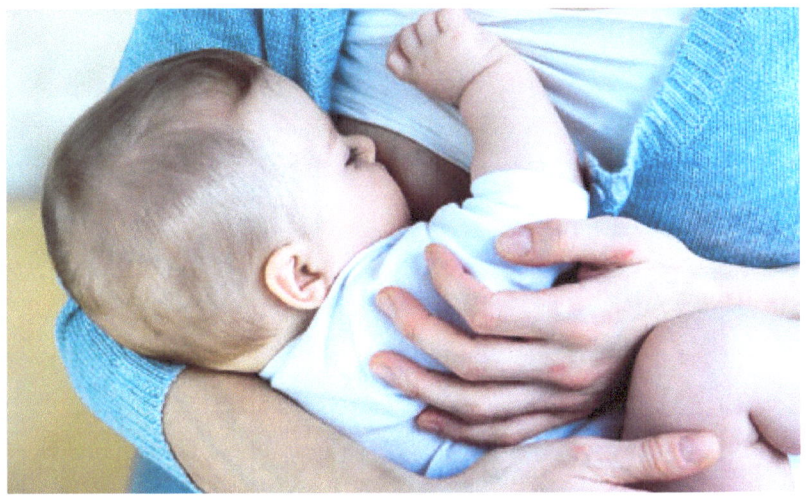

While it is an unpopular position within the breastfeeding community, the diet of the mother clearly impacts the quality of her breast milk (fats, vitamins and minerals in breast milk vary considerably based on the mother's diet although protein and immunoglobulins do not) and studies such as the Chinese Breast milk Study confirm this. Suggesting that a lactating mother can eat whatever she wants and still produce quality breast milk is also irresponsible and defies all common sense and historical study of healthy traditional cultures which put great emphasis on the quality of the diet of nursing mothers.

Generally speaking, a constipated baby that is breastfed is going to have a mother with gut dysbiosis issues, which means that she has an imbalanced gut herself and likely suffers from symptoms like constipation, gas, reflux, bloating, heartburn, IBS, ulcerative colitis or even skin issues such as eczema or psoriasis.

How to remedy a nursing mother's gut issues and thereby help her constipated baby? Well, there isn't an easy answer to this question, but no doubt, getting off of all processed foods and eating a minimal amount of grain based carbohydrates that are traditionally prepared would likely help tremendously. Going completely off grains is not a good idea as grains, particularly soaked cereal gruels, are known historically to encourage ample milk supply, so continuing to eat them in moderation is wise during lactation.

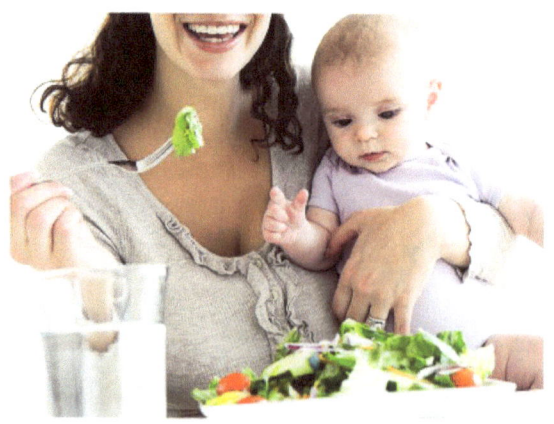

Elimination of pasteurized dairy and processed wheat would be a good first step if you are a breastfeeding mother with a constipated baby. I remember when I was nursing my child and he would spit up for an entire day and sometimes two days if I ate any processed wheat at all. The wheat I carefully prepared at home with fresh flour that was either soaked or sprouted did not give him any issues at all.

The bottom line if you are breastfeeding and have a constipated baby is to look to improve your diet and you will likely find your baby will have easier digestion and greater ease passing stools. And, once you wean, consider the GAPS Diet as a way to heal your gut once and for all so that your next baby doesn't have the same digestive issues when breastfeeding

6. Home Made Formula

It's no surprise that babies fed commercial formula can tend toward constipation due to the worrisome ingredients that make up these products. Commercial milk based baby formulas are, simply put, dangerous concoctions of denatured milk proteins and rancid vegetable oils which do a number on a baby's digestive system. Even the organic dairy formulas are not a wise choice as the violent processing is similar even if the ingredients are not as toxic. Hypoallergenic formulas are even worse as they contain an endocrine disrupting quantity of soy isoflavones that has the very real potential to damage your child's delicate and developing hormonal system.

The good news is that it is possible to make a nourishing formula for your baby yourself at home with quality ingredients that you source yourself (see Appendix 1). In a good share of cases, the simple act of switching baby off commercial formulas and onto a nourishing and much more digestible homemade formula will resolve the constipation issue.

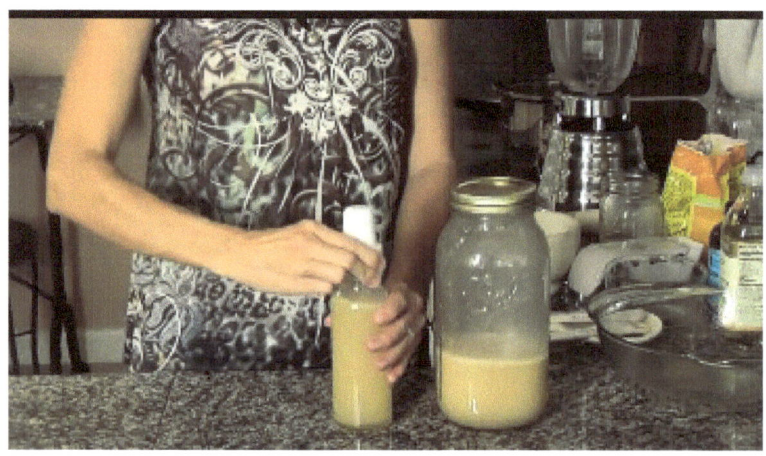

Try several small feedings offered more frequently throughout the day. By spreading out the feedings in this manner, your baby's digestive system has a better opportunity to digest the intake of formula. Keep track of how much you are feeding your baby in a 24 hour period and keep a count of the number of wet diaper changes. Try to decipher the amount of saturation of each diaper. There is a direct correlation to the intake of formula and the output of urine that your health care provider may need to know.

7. Adjusting Solid Food Diet

Certain types of solid food are more likely to trigger constipation, while the addition of other foods can prevent infant constipation. Decrease the amount of bananas and cooked carrots you provide the baby. These foods can cause or worsen constipation. Add more prunes, pears and apricots to the baby's diet. You can serve these foods by themselves in purees, or mix purees into the baby's cereal.

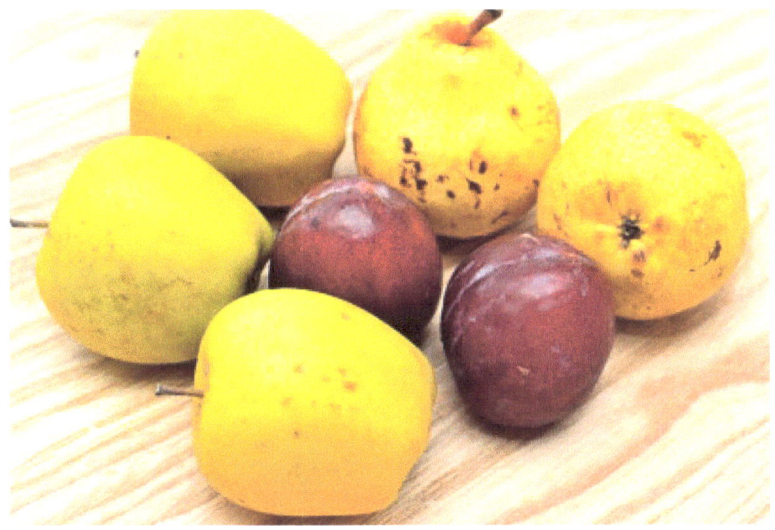

Puree some peas, spinach, or broccoli with a little water and feed to your new-born after they reach the age of 6 months. These green vegetables contain fibre which promotes gastrointestinal health. They will keep your baby on a regular cycle so that they don't end up getting constipated. Remember to keep the baby's foods varied to provide a balanced diet, and never force your baby to eat food if they do not want to. If you do, it can turn mealtimes into a battle and your child may start to think of eating as a negative and stressful experience.

One final suggestion is to avoid feeding baby any grain based foods in the first year of life. Amylase, the enzyme necessary to digest carbohydrates, is produced in only small amounts by a baby's digestive system before age one and so following a conventional doctor's advice to put rice cereal in a baby bottle (to encourage the child to sleep through the night) or feeding the child rice cereal as a first food is incredibly misguided and a potential disaster for a baby's developing gut environment.

Also, if the baby is eating any refined grains such as Cheerios, teething biscuits etc. (many Moms start these foods as soon as the child is sitting unassisted around 6 months) these should be stopped as these contribute to gut imbalance and perhaps constipation. No bread rolls or salad crackers for baby to chew on while in a high chair at a restaurant either!

If you are looking for an ideal early food, gelatine from homemade bone broths is incredibly soothing to a baby's digestive tract and is very nourishing as opposed to those indigestible grain based foods. Frequent gelatine in the diet goes a long way toward helping to resolve constipation issues.

8. Natural Oil Laxative

A healthy alternative to mineral oil is flax oil, which not only has laxative properties, but is a valuable source of omega 3 fats as well. (Although you may hear that mineral oil is a good oil to relieve constipation, because it is a mixture of hydrocarbons dried from petroleum products, I have never been convinced of its safety. And, unlike flax oil, it certainly has no nutritional benefits.)

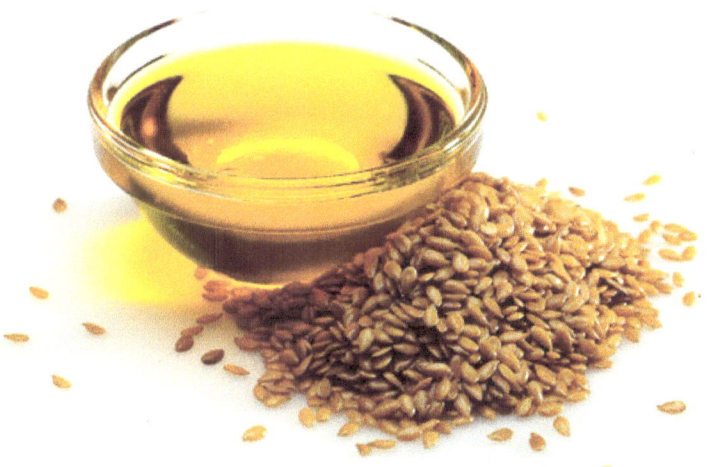

Unlike mineral oil, which slides through the intestines, possibly taking vitamins with it, flax oil is a nutrient that facilitates absorption of the vitamins.

Dosage of flax oil:

Infants: one teaspoon a day

Toddlers: two teaspoons a day

9. Baby Enema

To administer an enema to a baby, lubricate the tip of a bulb syringe with olive oil. Insert the tip of the bulb syringe into your baby's rectum ½ inches. The bulb should contain approximately 1 to 3 tablespoons of lukewarm water.

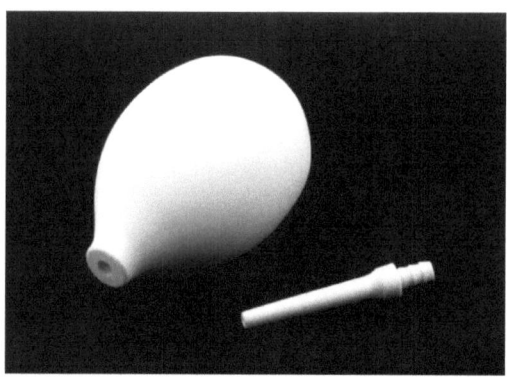

Gently squeeze the water into the colon. Assure that only the water goes into the colon, not any air that might be in the bulb. Wait a few minutes for your baby to pass a stool. Repeat this process if necessary.

10. Consult a Paediatrician

If the baby experiences persistent and severe constipation that is not affected by dietary or activity level adjustments, a doctor can assess whether there are any underlying causes for the constipation.

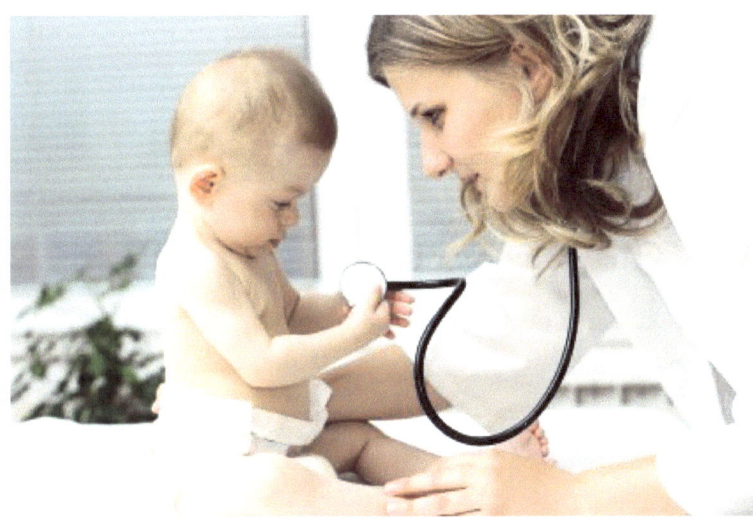

Understand that continual bouts of constipation can lead to other complications. The formation of haemorrhoids can become a potential risk when a constant strain on the sphincter muscles recurs. Anal fissures become another possibility with recurrent straining. Anal fissures will require a surgical procedure to treat them. Although generally associated with adults, small babies can develop these conditions as well if excessive constipation occurs.

Know that excessive straining can lead to a condition known as rectal prolapse. A small amount of the intestinal lining becomes forced out of the anus with the excessive and continuous straining efforts.

Consider the other complications that can occur with recurrent infant constipation. Faecal incontinence, rectal hernia and rectal bleeding are all characteristics of chronic constipation.

Understand that in severe cases, faecal impaction can occur. The course of action when faecal impaction occurs will be the administration of a mineral to aid in the softening of the stool. Removing the stool will be accomplished by the insertion of a finger into the anus to remove the stool manually.

Five Common Myths about Treating Infant Constipation

1. Glycerine Suppository

This could be useful at the outset to get that first stool moving, but even doctors discourage its regular use. A small amount of water inserted into the colon with an infant bulb syringe is just as effective and healthier.

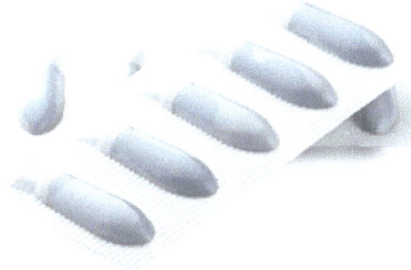

2. Karo syrup

Sugar in any form is not healthy for babies!

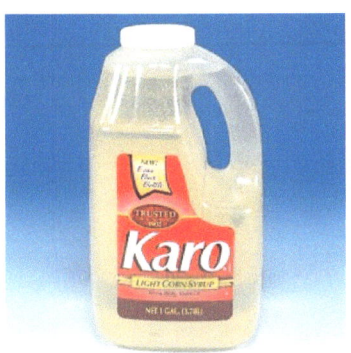

3. Mineral Oil

This is a mixture of hydrocarbons dried from petroleum products. It is not safe. It has no nutritional benefits. This oil can interfere with vitamin absorption.

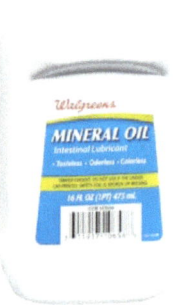

4. Fruit Juice

Many encourage parents to use fruit juice when an infant or toddler is constipated. I believe that babies, as well as adults, should limit the amount of juice that they drink as this can lead to all sorts of over consumption of sugar problems.

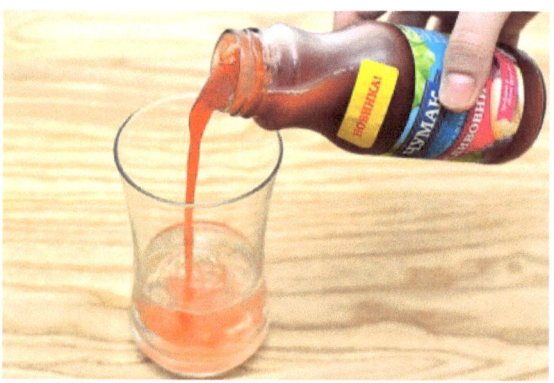

Too much juice can cause tummy aches, tooth decay, and perhaps obesity. In addition, kids can fill up on juice and miss other important sources of nutrition. Even the American Academy of Paediatrics issued recommendations in May 2001 to limit the amount of fruit juice for children.

5. Iron-Fortified Formulas

Before rushing to attribute your baby's constipation to the iron in the formula, you may be interested to know that controlled studies performed by the late Dr. Frank Oski, Professor and Chairman of the Department of Paediatrics at John Hopkins Medical School, showed that iron-fortified formulas do not cause constipation any more than formulas without iron.

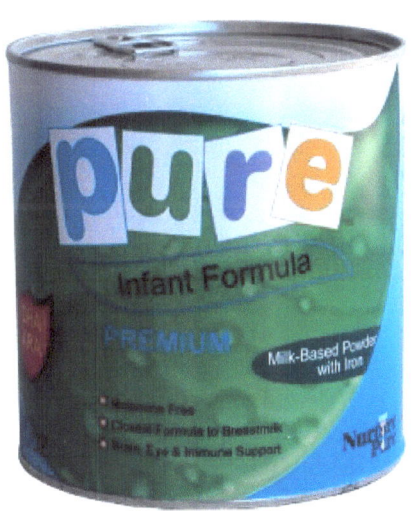

Appendix 1: Homemade Formula Recipes

Milk-Based Formula: Makes 36 ounces

Ingredients

2 cups whole milk, preferably unprocessed milk from pasture-fed cows

1/4 cup homemade liquid whey (See recipe for whey, below)

4 tablespoons lactose*

1 teaspoon bifidobacteriuminfntis**

2 or more tablespoons good quality cream (not ultra-pasteurized), more if you are using milk from Holstein cows

1 teaspoon regular dose cod liver oil or 1/2 teaspoon high-vitamin cod liver oil*

1 teaspoon expeller-expressed sunflower oil*

1 teaspoon extra virgin olive oil*

2 teaspoons coconut oil*

2 teaspoons Frontier brand nutritional yeast flakes*

2 teaspoons gelatine*

1 7/8 cups filtered water

1/4 teaspoon acerola powder*

Available from Radiant Life 888-593-8333

**Available from Natren 800-992-3323 or Radiant Life 888-593-8333*

Preparation

Add gelatine to water and heat gently until gelatine is dissolved. Place all ingredients in a very clean glass or stainless steel container and mix well. To serve, pour 6 to 8 ounces into a very clean glass bottle*, attach nipple and set in a pan of simmering water.

Heat until warm but not hot to the touch, shake bottle well and feed baby. (Never, never heat formula in a microwave oven!)

Variation: Goat Milk Formula

Although goat milk is rich in fat, it must be used with caution in infant feeding as it lacks folic acid and is low in vitamin B12, both of which are essential to the growth and development of the infant. Inclusion of nutritional yeast to provide folic acid is essential.

To compensate for low levels of vitamin B12, if preparing the Milk-Based Formula (above) with goat's milk, add 2 teaspoons frozen organic raw chicken liver, finely grated to the batch of formula.

Homemade Whey: Makes about 5 cups

Homemade whey is easy to make from good quality plain yoghurt, or from raw or cultured milk. You will need a large strainer that rests over a bowl. Line the strainer with a clean linen kitchen towel or several layers of cheesecloth.

If you are using yoghurt, place 2 quarts in the strainer lined with a tea towel. Cover with a plate and leave at room temperature overnight. The whey will drip out into the bowl. Place whey in clean glass jars and store in the refrigerator.

If you are using raw or cultured milk, place 2 quarts of the milk in a glass container and leave at room temperature for 2-4 days until the milk separates into curds and whey. Pour into the strainer lined with a tea towel and cover with a plate. Leave at room temperature overnight. The whey will drip out into the bowl. Store in clean glass jars in the refrigerator.

Liver-Based Formula: Makes 36 ounces

This liver-based formula also mimics the nutrient profile of mother's milk. It is extremely important to include coconut oil in this formula as it is the only ingredient that provides the special medium-chain saturated fats found in mother's milk.

Ingredients

3 3/4 cups homemade beef or chicken broth

2 ounces organic liver, cut into small pieces

5 tablespoons lactose*

1 teaspoon bifidobacteriuminfantis**

1/4 cup homemade liquid whey (See recipe for whey, below)

1 tablespoon coconut oil*

1 teaspoon cod liver oil or 1/2 teaspoon high-vitamin cod liver oil*

1 teaspoon unrefined sunflower oil*

2 teaspoons extra virgin olive oil

1 teaspoon acerola powder*

Preparation

Simmer liver gently in broth until the meat is cooked through. Liquefy using a handheld blender or in a food processor. When the liver broth has cooled, stir in remaining ingredients. Store in a very clean glass or stainless steel container.

To serve, stir formula well and pour 6 to 8 ounces in a very clean glass bottle. Attach a clean nipple and set in a pan of simmering water until formula is warm but not hot to the touch, shake well and feed to baby. (Never heat formula in a microwave oven!)

Appendix 2: Resource Guide

Useful Websites and Blogs

http://www.babycenter.com

http://www.webmd.com/parenting

http://www.mayoclinic.com/health

http://www.askdrsears.com/topics/childhood-illnesses/constipation

http://www.babycures.com

http://www.justmommies.com

http://www.netmums.com

http://pregnant.thebump.com

http://www.circleofmoms.com

www.ingramcontent.com/pod-product-compliance
Lightning Source LLC
Chambersburg PA
CBHW050849290526
45792CB00002B/581